The Pandemic Paradox: Achieving Work-Life Equilibrium for Everyone

Sahil Singh

Copyright © [2023]

Title: The Pandemic Paradox: Achieving Work-Life Equilibrium for Everyone

Author's: Sahil Singh.

All rights reserved. No part of this publication may be reproduced, stored in a retrieval system, or transmitted in any form or by any means, electronic, mechanical, photocopying, recording, or otherwise, without the prior written permission of the publisher or author, except in the case of brief quotations embodied in critical reviews and certain other non-commercial uses permitted by copyright law.

This book was printed and published by [Publisher's: Sahil Singh] in [2023]

ISBN:

TABLE OF CONTENTS

Chapter 1: The Pandemic Paradox: Understanding the Work-Life Equilibrium Challenge   08

The Shift to Remote Work: A New Reality

The sudden transition to remote work

The benefits and challenges of working from home

Redefining the traditional work-life balance

The Impact of the Pandemic on Personal Life

Strains on personal relationships and family dynamics

Emotional and mental health challenges

Coping mechanisms and self-care during uncertain times

Chapter 2: Balancing Work and Personal Life: Strategies for Success   24

Establishing Boundaries for a Productive Workday

Creating a designated workspace at home

Setting clear work hours and avoiding burnout

Communicating boundaries with colleagues, employers, and family

Time Management Techniques for Efficiency and Fulfillment

Prioritizing tasks and setting realistic goals

Implementing effective time-blocking strategies

Maximizing productivity by minimizing distractions

Nurturing Relationships and Personal Connections

Maintaining social connections while physically distant

Strengthening relationships with loved ones

Investing time in self-reflection and personal growth

Chapter 3: Overcoming Challenges and Adapting to Change 48

Overcoming Remote Work Challenges

Managing isolation and loneliness

Overcoming technological barriers and connectivity issues

Building a virtual support network

Embracing Flexibility and Resilience

Adapting to changing work demands and expectations

Embracing a growth mindset and embracing opportunities for learning

Resilience-building practices to cope with uncertainty

Chapter 4: Creating a Culture of Work-Life Equilibrium   64

Employer Responsibility: Fostering Work-Life Balance

Implementing flexible work policies and practices

Promoting employee well-being and mental health support

Encouraging work-life integration rather than separation

The Importance of Self-Advocacy in Achieving Equilibrium

Communicating personal needs and boundaries effectively

Negotiating work arrangements and accommodations

Empowering individuals to prioritize their well-being

Chapter 5: Thriving in the New Normal: Sustaining Work-Life Equilibrium 80

Embracing a Hybrid Work Model

Balancing remote and in-person work arrangements

Leveraging technology for efficient collaboration

Reaping the benefits of a flexible work environment

The Future of Work-Life Equilibrium

Long-term strategies for maintaining equilibrium post-pandemic

Recognizing the evolving needs of a diverse workforce

Advocating for a sustainable work-life equilibrium for everyone

Conclusion: Achieving Work-Life Equilibrium: A Journey of Balance and Growth 97

Chapter 1: The Pandemic Paradox: Understanding the Work-Life Equilibrium Challenge

The Shift to Remote Work: A New Reality

In recent times, the world has witnessed an unprecedented shift in the way we work. The COVID-19 pandemic has forced organizations and individuals to adapt quickly to a new reality – remote work. This subchapter delves into the implications of this shift and provides valuable insights on how to be productive during these challenging times.

Remote work has become a necessity in order to maintain business continuity and ensure the safety of employees. While it may seem daunting at first, it presents a unique opportunity to redefine the way we approach work and achieve a better work-life equilibrium. Gone are the days of long commutes, rigid schedules, and limited flexibility. Remote work allows us to create a more balanced lifestyle, where we can allocate time for personal and professional pursuits more efficiently.

To be productive during this pandemic and in a remote work environment, it is crucial to establish a routine. Setting clear boundaries between work and personal life is essential. Designate a dedicated workspace, preferably away from distractions, to create a focused environment. Establish a schedule that aligns with your personal preferences and work requirements. This will help maintain a sense of normalcy and structure, enhancing productivity and overall well-being.

Communication is key in a remote work setup. Regularly engage with your team through virtual meetings, instant messaging, or video conferences. Foster open and transparent communication channels to ensure that everyone is on the same page and that collaboration remains strong. Additionally, leverage technology tools and platforms to streamline workflows, manage tasks, and track progress effectively.

Finding a balance between work and personal life is crucial for maintaining productivity and avoiding burnout. Take regular breaks, practice self-care, and prioritize your well-being. Engage in activities that bring you joy, exercise regularly, and maintain a healthy work-life integration.

While the shift to remote work may have been sudden, it offers a unique opportunity for personal growth. Use this time to develop new skills, enhance your knowledge, and explore new interests. Invest in your professional development through online courses, webinars, or virtual conferences. This will not only make you more valuable in the marketplace but also boost your confidence and job satisfaction.

In conclusion, the shift to remote work is a new reality that has its challenges but also presents immense opportunities. By establishing a routine, maintaining clear communication, prioritizing well-being, and investing in personal growth, we can navigate this new landscape and achieve a harmonious work-life equilibrium. Embrace this change, adapt to it, and thrive in the face of adversity.

The sudden transition to remote work

The sudden transition to remote work has become one of the most significant and unexpected changes brought about by the ongoing pandemic. As offices shuttered and employees were faced with the reality of working from their homes, it was clear that this was not just a temporary adjustment but a new way of life for many. This subchapter aims to explore the challenges and opportunities that come with this sudden shift and provide practical insights on how to be productive during these trying times.

For many individuals, the initial transition to remote work was a shock to their system. The lines between work and personal life became blurred, creating new challenges in finding a balance between the two. Distractions at home, lack of structure, and the absence of a dedicated workspace posed obstacles to productivity. However, with the right mindset and strategies, it is possible to not only adapt but thrive in this new work landscape.

First and foremost, it is crucial to establish a routine and maintain a sense of structure. Designating a specific workspace, setting regular working hours, and adhering to a schedule can help create a sense of normalcy and increase productivity. Additionally, taking breaks and incorporating physical activity into the day can help alleviate stress and improve focus.

Technology has played a pivotal role in enabling remote work, but it also presents its own set of challenges. Distractions such as social media, emails, and constant notifications can hinder productivity. Setting boundaries with technology, such as establishing specific times for checking emails and silencing non-essential notifications, can help combat these distractions and maintain focus on the task at hand.

Furthermore, effective communication and collaboration with colleagues are vital for remote work success. Utilizing video conferencing tools, instant messaging platforms, and project management software can help bridge the physical gap and foster teamwork. Regular check-ins and clear communication channels are essential to ensure that everyone is on the same page and working towards common goals.

While the sudden transition to remote work may have been unexpected, it also presents unique opportunities. This subchapter will delve into strategies for leveraging the flexibility and autonomy that remote work offers to enhance productivity and achieve a better work-life equilibrium.

In conclusion, the sudden transition to remote work has undoubtedly posed numerous challenges for individuals striving to be productive during the pandemic. However, by implementing effective strategies and embracing the opportunities that remote work presents, it is possible to achieve a sense of equilibrium and thrive in this new work landscape.

The benefits and challenges of working from home

In recent times, the concept of working from home has gained significant attention, thanks to the unprecedented circumstances brought about by the global pandemic. As the world grapples with the challenges posed by the COVID-19 outbreak, individuals from all walks of life have been forced to adapt to a new normal – working remotely.

The benefits of working from home are numerous and extend beyond the realm of convenience. One of the most prominent advantages is the flexibility it offers. Without the need to commute to an office, employees can save precious time and redirect it towards more productive activities. This newfound freedom allows for a better work-life balance, enabling individuals to spend quality time with their families, pursue hobbies, or engage in self-care practices.

Moreover, working from home eliminates the distractions often encountered in a traditional office setting. Employees can create personalized workspaces suited to their preferences, resulting in increased focus and productivity. The absence of unnecessary meetings and water-cooler conversations can significantly boost efficiency, allowing tasks to be completed in a shorter time span.

For many, the financial benefits of working from home are also significant. Individuals can save on transportation costs, expensive work attire, and daily lunches, resulting in considerable savings over time. Additionally, the reduced need for office space can be advantageous for employers, as it leads to reduced overhead costs.

However, remote work is not without its challenges. One of the primary obstacles is establishing clear boundaries between work and personal life. With the office now just a few steps away, it can be tempting to blur the lines and work longer hours. This can lead to burnout and hamper one's overall well-being. Therefore, it becomes crucial to set strict schedules and adhere to them, ensuring that personal time is respected and protected.

Another challenge is the potential for isolation and decreased social interaction. Working from home can limit opportunities for face-to-face communication and collaboration, which can impact team dynamics and creativity. To combat this, it is essential to utilize suitable digital tools and platforms for effective communication and maintain regular check-ins with colleagues.

In conclusion, the benefits of working from home during a pandemic are undeniable. It offers flexibility, increased productivity, financial savings, and a better work-life balance. However, it is essential to navigate the challenges that come with remote work, such as maintaining boundaries and combating isolation. By acknowledging these challenges and implementing strategies to overcome them, individuals can successfully achieve work-life equilibrium during these uncertain times.

Redefining the traditional work-life balance

In the wake of the global pandemic, our lives have been upended in unimaginable ways. The way we work, live, and engage with the world has undergone a seismic shift, forcing us to redefine what work-life balance truly means. In this subchapter, we will explore the new paradigm of work-life equilibrium and how it can be achieved for everyone, particularly in the context of being productive during a pandemic.

Gone are the days when work-life balance simply meant separating our professional and personal lives. The lines between these two realms have become increasingly blurred, as our homes have transformed into makeshift offices and our personal responsibilities intertwine with our professional obligations. However, this new reality presents an opportunity for us to revolutionize our approach to work and life.

The concept of work-life equilibrium emphasizes the integration and harmony of these two spheres, rather than their strict separation. It recognizes that the traditional 9-to-5 work model may not be the most effective or fulfilling way to navigate the current landscape. Instead, it encourages individuals to find a rhythm that suits their unique circumstances, allowing for flexibility, adaptability, and holistic self-care.

To achieve work-life equilibrium during a pandemic, it is crucial to prioritize self-care and well-being. This means setting boundaries and carving out time for rest, relaxation, and leisure activities. Engaging in hobbies, practicing mindfulness, and fostering connections with loved ones can help maintain a sense of balance and prevent burnout.

Additionally, embracing remote work and leveraging technology can be powerful tools in achieving work-life equilibrium. Working from home offers newfound flexibility, allowing individuals to tailor their schedules to optimize productivity and personal fulfillment. Embracing digital platforms for collaboration and communication can also foster a sense of connection and engagement, mitigating the potential isolation that may arise from remote work.

Moreover, organizations need to play an active role in redefining work-life balance for their employees. They should cultivate a culture that values work-life equilibrium, providing resources and support for employees to thrive in both their personal and professional lives. Offering flexible work arrangements, promoting work-life integration, and encouraging open communication can create an environment that promotes well-being and productivity.

In conclusion, redefining the traditional work-life balance is crucial in the midst of a pandemic. Embracing the concept of work-life equilibrium allows us to navigate this uncertain territory with resilience and purpose. By prioritizing self-care, embracing remote work, and fostering supportive organizational cultures, we can achieve a harmonious integration of work and life that benefits everyone. Let us seize this opportunity to forge a new path towards work-life equilibrium, where productivity and well-being go hand in hand.

The Impact of the Pandemic on Personal Life

The COVID-19 pandemic has had a profound impact on every aspect of our lives, including our personal lives. From the sudden shift to remote work to the isolation caused by social distancing measures, the pandemic has forced us to adapt and find new ways to navigate our daily routines. In this subchapter, we will explore the various ways the pandemic has affected our personal lives and discuss strategies for maintaining productivity during these challenging times.

One of the most significant impacts of the pandemic on personal life has been the blurring of boundaries between work and home. With remote work becoming the new norm, many individuals find themselves struggling to separate work obligations from personal responsibilities. This constant overlap can lead to burnout and decreased productivity. To overcome this challenge, it is crucial to establish clear boundaries and create a dedicated workspace within your home. Setting specific work hours and taking regular breaks can help maintain a healthy work-life balance.

Moreover, the pandemic has also brought feelings of isolation and loneliness. Social distancing measures have limited our ability to interact with friends and family, leading to increased feelings of loneliness and anxiety. It is important to prioritize self-care during these times by engaging in activities that bring you joy and connecting with loved ones virtually. Scheduling regular video calls or virtual gatherings can help combat feelings of isolation and keep relationships strong.

Additionally, the pandemic has disrupted our usual routines and activities, making it difficult to stay motivated and focused. Developing a new routine and setting achievable goals can help combat this lack of motivation. This could include incorporating regular exercise, practicing mindfulness, and exploring new hobbies. By setting small, attainable goals, you can maintain a sense of purpose and productivity during these uncertain times.

In conclusion, the pandemic has undeniably had a significant impact on our personal lives. From blurring work-life boundaries to feelings of isolation and disrupted routines, it is essential to acknowledge and address these challenges. By establishing clear boundaries, prioritizing self-care, and setting achievable goals, we can strive for a sense of productivity and fulfillment even in the midst of a pandemic. Remember, we are all in this together, and by supporting one another, we can navigate these unprecedented times with resilience and strength.

Strains on personal relationships and family dynamics

In the midst of a global pandemic, our lives have undergone significant changes, impacting every aspect of our existence. From the way we work to how we interact with our loved ones, the pandemic has introduced new challenges and strains on personal relationships and family dynamics. In this subchapter, we will explore the various ways the pandemic has affected our interpersonal connections and provide insights on how to navigate these challenges while maintaining productivity.

One of the most notable challenges we face during this time is the blurring of boundaries between work and personal life. As remote work becomes the norm, many individuals find themselves working longer hours, often encroaching on their personal time. This strain can lead to increased stress, decreased productivity, and ultimately, strained relationships with family members. It is crucial to establish clear boundaries, communicate openly with loved ones about work expectations, and prioritize quality time together.

Moreover, the pandemic has forced families to adapt to new routines and roles. With schools and daycares closed or operating under limited capacity, parents have taken on the additional role of educators while juggling their own work responsibilities. This shift in dynamics can create tensions and conflicts within the family unit. To alleviate these strains, it is essential to foster open communication, share responsibilities, and establish a flexible schedule that accommodates both work and family commitments.

Additionally, the lack of social interactions and physical distancing measures have taken a toll on our mental and emotional well-being. Human beings are social creatures, and the absence of regular social connections can lead to feelings of isolation and loneliness. This emotional strain can impact our ability to be productive and can also put a strain on personal relationships. It is vital to prioritize self-care, maintain virtual connections with friends and family, and seek professional help if needed.

In conclusion, the pandemic has undoubtedly brought about strains on personal relationships and family dynamics. However, by recognizing and addressing these challenges, we can achieve a sense of work-life equilibrium. By setting boundaries, fostering open communication, sharing responsibilities, and prioritizing self-care and social connections, we can navigate these turbulent times while maintaining productivity and cultivating healthy relationships. Remember, we are all in this together, and by supporting one another, we can overcome the challenges and emerge stronger as individuals and as families.

Emotional and mental health challenges

Emotional and Mental Health Challenges: Navigating Through the Pandemic

In these unprecedented times, the COVID-19 pandemic has brought about numerous challenges that have affected almost every aspect of our lives. From the way we work to how we interact with others, the pandemic has created a new normal that has significantly impacted our emotional and mental well-being. In this subchapter, we will explore the various challenges we face and provide strategies to help us maintain emotional and mental health during these uncertain times.

One of the major challenges we encounter is the feeling of isolation and loneliness. With social distancing measures in place, many of us are physically separated from our loved ones, friends, and colleagues. This lack of social interaction can take a toll on our emotional well-being. However, it is essential to remember that we are not alone in this situation. Connecting virtually with others through video calls, online communities, and social media platforms can help alleviate feelings of isolation and provide a sense of belonging.

Another significant challenge is the increased stress and anxiety caused by the pandemic. The fear of contracting the virus, financial worries, and uncertainty about the future can all contribute to heightened stress levels. To manage these challenges, it is crucial to prioritize self-care and establish healthy coping mechanisms. Engaging in activities that bring joy and relaxation, such as meditation, exercise, or pursuing hobbies, can help reduce stress and improve mental well-being.

Moreover, the blurring of boundaries between work and personal life during the pandemic has led to challenges in maintaining a productive mindset. With remote work becoming the new norm for many, it can be challenging to separate work life from personal life, resulting in burnout and decreased productivity. Setting clear boundaries, creating a dedicated workspace, and establishing a daily routine can help maintain a healthy work-life balance and increase productivity.

Additionally, the constant exposure to news and information about the pandemic can be overwhelming and contribute to anxiety. It is essential to limit our exposure to negative news and seek information from reliable sources. Practicing mindfulness and focusing on the present moment can also help alleviate stress and anxiety related to uncertain future events.

In conclusion, the emotional and mental health challenges brought on by the pandemic are widespread and affect us all. However, by recognizing and addressing these challenges, we can navigate through these uncertain times. Prioritizing self-care, maintaining social connections, establishing boundaries, and practicing mindfulness are all crucial strategies to maintain emotional and mental well-being. By taking these steps, we can achieve a sense of equilibrium and resilience, enabling us to navigate the pandemic and emerge stronger on the other side. Remember, we are all in this together, and together, we can overcome these challenges.

Coping mechanisms and self-care during uncertain times

Introduction

In times of uncertainty and crisis, it is essential to develop effective coping mechanisms and prioritize self-care. The COVID-19 pandemic has brought unprecedented challenges, disrupting our daily lives and blurring the line between work and personal life. In this subchapter, we will explore strategies to maintain productivity and well-being during these uncertain times, ensuring a healthy work-life equilibrium for everyone.

1. Establish a Routine

Creating a structured routine can provide a sense of normalcy and stability amidst chaos. Set a consistent wake-up time, allocate specific hours for work, breaks, exercise, and leisure activities. This helps maintain a healthy work-life balance and prevents burnout.

2. Set Realistic Goals

During a pandemic, it is important to acknowledge that circumstances have changed. Set realistic goals and prioritize tasks that align with your current situation. Be flexible and adapt to the new normal, allowing yourself room for adjustments and self-compassion.

3. Embrace Remote Work

Remote work has become the norm for many during the pandemic. Embrace this opportunity by creating a designated workspace, minimizing distractions, and establishing boundaries between work and personal life. Set aside time for breaks, physical activity, and social interaction to combat the isolation that remote work may bring.

4. Practice Mindfulness and Stress Management

In uncertain times, it is crucial to take care of your mental well-being. Engage in mindfulness practices, such as meditation or deep breathing exercises, to reduce stress and anxiety. Be aware of your emotions and seek professional help if needed. Stay connected with loved ones through virtual platforms, fostering social support and reducing feelings of isolation.

5. Prioritize Self-Care Activities

Make self-care a priority during uncertain times. Engage in activities that bring you joy and relaxation, such as reading, taking baths, listening to music, or pursuing hobbies. Prioritize sleep, exercise regularly, and maintain a healthy diet. Remember, self-care is not selfish but essential for overall well-being.

Conclusion

The COVID-19 pandemic has undoubtedly created a unique set of challenges for everyone. By implementing coping mechanisms and practicing self-care, we can navigate these uncertain times with resilience and achieve a healthy work-life equilibrium. Remember to establish routines, set realistic goals, embrace remote work, practice mindfulness, and prioritize self-care activities. Let us come together as a community, supporting one another, and emerging stronger from this pandemic.

Chapter 2: Balancing Work and Personal Life: Strategies for Success

Establishing Boundaries for a Productive Workday

In the midst of the ongoing pandemic, maintaining a productive workday has become a challenge for many individuals. The blurred lines between work and personal life have made it difficult to find a balance and prevent burnout. However, by establishing clear boundaries, you can create a productive workday that allows you to maintain your mental well-being and achieve a work-life equilibrium.

One of the first steps in establishing boundaries for a productive workday is creating a designated workspace. Whether it's a separate room or a specific area in your home, having a dedicated space for work can help you maintain focus and productivity. When you step into this workspace, your mind automatically switches to work mode, eliminating distractions and increasing your efficiency.

Another crucial aspect of boundary-setting is defining your working hours. With remote work becoming the norm, it's easy to let work bleed into your personal time. However, setting specific working hours and sticking to them ensures that you have time for both work and personal activities. Communicate these hours with your colleagues and establish a routine that allows you to be fully present during your working hours and disconnect once they are over.

Additionally, it's vital to establish boundaries with technology. Constant notifications from emails, messages, and social media can disrupt your focus and hinder your productivity. Consider setting specific times to check and respond to emails or messages, rather than being constantly available. By creating this boundary, you can allocate uninterrupted time to focus on your tasks and reduce the temptation to multitask.

Moreover, boundaries should also extend to your personal life. It's important to set aside time for self-care, hobbies, and quality time with loved ones. By scheduling and prioritizing these activities, you can recharge and avoid burnout, ultimately enhancing your overall productivity.

Remember, everyone's boundaries may differ, so it's essential to find what works best for you. Experiment with different strategies and evaluate their effectiveness. Regularly reassess and adjust your boundaries as needed to ensure they align with your goals and well-being.

By establishing boundaries for a productive workday, you can strike a balance between work and personal life, even during the pandemic. These boundaries will not only enhance your productivity but also contribute to your mental and emotional well-being. So, take the necessary steps today and create a workday that allows you to thrive in both your professional and personal pursuits.

Creating a designated workspace at home

In the midst of the pandemic, many of us have found ourselves navigating the challenges of working from home. Whether you're a parent juggling childcare and professional responsibilities or an individual adapting to a new remote work setup, creating a designated workspace at home is essential for maintaining productivity and achieving work-life equilibrium.

A designated workspace provides structure and helps to separate your personal and professional life, even if they're now occurring under the same roof. To establish an effective workspace, consider the following tips:

1. Find a Quiet Corner: Identify a space in your home that is relatively free from distractions. This could be a spare room, a corner in your living room, or even a cozy nook under the stairs. Choose a spot that allows you to focus and minimizes interruptions.

2. Invest in Ergonomic Furniture: Working from home often means spending long hours seated at a desk. Invest in an ergonomic chair and desk to ensure proper support for your body and reduce the risk of developing discomfort or pain. Your physical well-being is crucial for maintaining productivity.

3. Organize and Declutter: A cluttered workspace can affect your ability to concentrate and think clearly. Take the time to declutter your designated area, ensuring that only essential items are within reach. Use storage solutions like shelves, drawers, or bins to keep everything organized and easily accessible.

4. Personalize Your Space: Make your designated workspace a pleasant environment by adding personal touches. Display photos, artwork, or motivational quotes that inspire you. Consider adding plants to bring nature indoors and create a calming atmosphere.

5. Establish Boundaries: Communicate with your household members about the importance of respecting your workspace and uninterrupted work hours. Set clear boundaries and establish a routine that allows you to focus on your tasks without distractions.

6. Minimize Digital Distractions: With the internet just a click away, it's easy to get sidetracked by social media or other online temptations. Use browser extensions or apps to block time-wasting websites during your work hours and establish designated break times for checking personal notifications.

Creating a designated workspace at home is a crucial step towards achieving work-life equilibrium during the pandemic. By following these tips, you can create an environment that supports productivity, focus, and a healthy work-life balance. Remember, everyone's situation is unique, so find what works best for you and adapt accordingly.

Setting clear work hours and avoiding burnout

In these unprecedented times, the COVID-19 pandemic has drastically transformed the way we work and live. Many of us have found ourselves juggling remote work, household chores, and caring for our loved ones, all within the confines of our homes. As a result, maintaining a healthy work-life balance has become more challenging than ever. However, by setting clear work hours and prioritizing our well-being, we can navigate this pandemic paradox and achieve work-life equilibrium.

One of the crucial steps towards achieving a healthy work-life balance during the pandemic is setting clear work hours. Without the physical separation of the office and the home, it is easy for work to seep into every aspect of our lives. By establishing a dedicated workspace and sticking to a consistent schedule, we can create boundaries between work and personal life. Communicating these boundaries with our colleagues, employers, and family members is essential to ensure everyone understands and respects our designated work hours.

Moreover, avoiding burnout is paramount for being productive during the pandemic. Recognizing our limitations and taking regular breaks throughout the day are vital to maintaining our mental and physical well-being. It is crucial to step away from our screens, engage in physical activity, and practice mindfulness or relaxation techniques. Prioritizing self-care activities, such as pursuing hobbies, spending time with loved ones, or simply taking time for ourselves, can help replenish our energy and prevent burnout.

Additionally, it is necessary to cultivate open communication with our employers and colleagues. If we are feeling overwhelmed or facing difficulties in managing our workload, it is important to express our concerns. Employers should seek to create a supportive work environment that encourages open dialogue and provides resources to help employees navigate the challenges of remote work.

In conclusion, setting clear work hours and avoiding burnout are crucial steps towards achieving work-life equilibrium during the pandemic. By establishing boundaries, taking regular breaks, and communicating effectively, we can maintain our productivity and well-being. It is important to remember that we are all navigating these challenging times together, and by prioritizing our mental and physical health, we can overcome the pandemic paradox and find balance in our lives.

Communicating boundaries with colleagues, employers, and family

In today's fast-paced and interconnected world, maintaining a healthy work-life balance can be challenging, especially during a pandemic. The lines between professional and personal life have become blurred, with remote work blurring the boundaries even further. However, it is essential to establish clear and effective communication boundaries with our colleagues, employers, and even family members to achieve a sense of equilibrium and maintain productivity during these unprecedented times.

When it comes to communicating boundaries with colleagues, it is crucial to establish expectations and guidelines from the start. Clearly communicate your working hours, preferred methods of communication, and availability. This will help reduce unnecessary interruptions and enable you to focus on your tasks. Similarly, encourage your colleagues to respect your boundaries and avoid contacting you during non-working hours, unless it's an emergency. By setting these boundaries, you can create a more conducive work environment and increase overall productivity.

When it comes to employers, open and honest communication is key. Discuss your needs and limitations with your employer, especially if you are juggling multiple responsibilities, such as childcare or eldercare during the pandemic. Negotiate a flexible schedule or alternative arrangements that can accommodate your personal obligations without compromising your professional commitments. Remember, employers are also navigating these challenging times, and open dialogue can lead to mutually beneficial solutions.

Communication boundaries with family members are equally important. Just because you are working from home does not mean you are available at all times. Explain to your family members the importance of undisturbed work hours and set clear expectations regarding interruptions during your designated work time. Establishing a dedicated workspace within your home can also help signal to your family members that you are in "work mode" and should not be disturbed unless absolutely necessary.

By effectively communicating boundaries with colleagues, employers, and family members, you can strike a balance between your personal and professional life during the pandemic. Remember that setting boundaries is not selfish; it is a way to protect your well-being and ensure that you can give your best in all aspects of life. Be open, clear, and assertive in your communication, and don't be afraid to recalibrate and adjust as needed. Together, we can navigate the challenges of the pandemic and achieve work-life equilibrium for everyone.

Time Management Techniques for Efficiency and Fulfillment

In the midst of the COVID-19 pandemic, many of us have found ourselves facing unprecedented challenges in managing our time effectively. Balancing work and personal life has become increasingly difficult as the boundaries between the two blur, leaving us feeling overwhelmed and unfulfilled. However, with the right time management techniques, we can regain control over our lives and achieve a sense of efficiency and fulfillment even in these uncertain times.

One of the most effective strategies for managing time during the pandemic is creating a daily schedule. Start by identifying your priorities and allocating specific time slots for each task. Be realistic about what you can accomplish in a given day and allow for flexibility to accommodate unexpected interruptions. Remember to include breaks throughout the day to recharge and maintain focus.

Another essential technique is setting clear boundaries between work and personal life. Working from home can easily lead to a blurring of these boundaries, causing work to spill into personal time and vice versa. Establishing a designated workspace and adhering to set working hours can help create a sense of structure and prevent burnout. Similarly, ensure that personal time is dedicated solely to activities that bring you joy and relaxation.

To enhance efficiency, consider implementing the Pomodoro Technique. This technique involves breaking work into 25-minute intervals, known as "pomodoros," followed by short breaks. After completing four pomodoros, take a longer break. This method helps maintain focus and prevents fatigue, allowing for greater productivity throughout the day.

Furthermore, it is crucial to prioritize self-care and maintain a healthy work-life balance. Engage in activities that promote physical and mental well-being, such as exercise, meditation, or hobbies. Remember that taking care of yourself is not a luxury but a necessity for productivity and fulfillment.

Utilizing technology and digital tools can also significantly aid in time management. Explore productivity apps and software that can help track your tasks, set reminders, and manage your schedule efficiently. Additionally, leverage communication and collaboration tools to streamline work processes and enhance productivity while working remotely.

In conclusion, the pandemic has presented us with unique challenges in managing our time effectively. By implementing these time management techniques, we can regain control over our lives, increase productivity, and find a sense of fulfillment. Remember to create a daily schedule, set clear boundaries, use the Pomodoro Technique, prioritize self-care, and leverage technology to optimize your time and achieve work-life equilibrium even during these uncertain times.

Prioritizing tasks and setting realistic goals

In these unprecedented times, maintaining productivity while navigating the challenges of a pandemic can be a daunting task. However, by prioritizing tasks and setting realistic goals, you can achieve a balance between work and personal life, ensuring a sense of equilibrium during these uncertain times.

When it comes to prioritizing tasks, it is crucial to identify what needs your immediate attention. Start by creating a to-do list and categorize tasks based on their urgency and importance. This will help you focus on essential responsibilities and avoid being overwhelmed by a long list of tasks. By prioritizing, you can allocate your time and energy more effectively, ensuring that you accomplish what truly matters.

Setting realistic goals is equally important. Understand that the circumstances we are currently living in have significantly impacted our lives and work dynamics. Therefore, it is crucial to adjust our expectations and set achievable goals. Be mindful of your limitations and consider the external factors that may affect your productivity. By setting attainable goals, you can maintain motivation and avoid feeling discouraged or burnt out.

Another useful practice is to break down larger goals into smaller, more manageable tasks. This approach not only helps you stay organized but also provides a sense of accomplishment as you complete each task. Celebrating these small victories can boost your morale and keep you motivated to tackle the next challenge.

During a pandemic, it is essential to strike a balance between work and personal life. Establish boundaries and allocate specific time slots for work-related activities, as well as personal activities and self-care. By doing so, you create a structured routine that helps you maintain focus while ensuring you have time to recharge and rejuvenate.

Remember, it is perfectly normal to face challenges and experience setbacks during these unprecedented times. Be kind to yourself and practice self-compassion. Adjust your expectations as needed and prioritize your mental and physical well-being. Seek support from loved ones or professional resources if necessary.

By prioritizing tasks and setting realistic goals, you can achieve a sense of work-life equilibrium even in the midst of a pandemic. Embrace flexibility and adaptability, and remember that taking care of yourself is just as important as achieving professional success. Together, we can navigate these challenging times and emerge stronger, more resilient, and balanced.

Implementing effective time-blocking strategies

In the midst of a global pandemic, achieving work-life equilibrium seems like an elusive goal for many individuals. With the lines between work and personal life increasingly blurred, it is crucial to adopt effective time-blocking strategies to optimize productivity and maintain a sense of balance. This subchapter explores various techniques that can help you make the most out of your time and navigate the challenges posed by the pandemic.

1. Prioritize and Plan: Start by identifying your most important tasks and setting realistic goals for each day. Consider both work-related and personal responsibilities to create a comprehensive plan. By establishing priorities, you can ensure that you allocate time for essential activities while avoiding overwhelm.

2. Create Time Blocks: Rather than allowing your day to unfold haphazardly, divide it into specific time blocks dedicated to different activities. This approach allows you to allocate focused time for work, personal chores, exercise, relaxation, and family time. Be sure to include breaks within your schedule to recharge and avoid burnout.

3. Set Boundaries: Working from home during the pandemic often blurs the boundaries between work and personal life. To overcome this challenge, establish clear boundaries by defining specific working hours and sticking to them. Communicate these boundaries to your colleagues and family members to ensure uninterrupted focus during work hours and uninterrupted personal time afterwards.

4. Eliminate Distractions: Minimize distractions that can hinder productivity by creating a dedicated workspace and turning off

notifications on your devices during work time. When you have designated time blocks for specific activities, commit fully to them, avoiding multitasking and maintaining a laser-like focus on the task at hand.

5. Review and Adjust: Regularly review your time-blocking strategies to assess their effectiveness. Identify any areas where adjustments are needed and make necessary changes to optimize your productivity and overall well-being. Remember, flexibility is key as you adapt to the ever-changing landscape of the pandemic.

By implementing these effective time-blocking strategies, you can regain control over your time and achieve a sense of work-life equilibrium. Embracing this approach will not only enhance your productivity but also enable you to nurture your personal life and well-being during these challenging times. Remember, we are all in this together, and by adopting these strategies, we can navigate the pandemic paradox and foster a better future for ourselves and everyone around us.

Maximizing productivity by minimizing distractions

In the midst of a global pandemic, maintaining productivity levels can be challenging for everyone. As we navigate through this new normal, it is crucial to find effective strategies to minimize distractions and optimize our work-life equilibrium. In this subchapter, we will explore various techniques to help you stay focused and productive during these unprecedented times.

One of the first steps in maximizing productivity is acknowledging the distractions that surround us. Whether it's the constant stream of notifications on our smartphones or the temptation to binge-watch our favorite shows, distractions can easily derail our progress. By identifying these distractions, we can take proactive measures to minimize their impact on our work.

Creating a dedicated workspace is essential for achieving productivity. This space should be separate from areas associated with relaxation or leisure activities. Clearing clutter and organizing your workspace can significantly enhance focus and reduce distractions. Additionally, establishing a daily routine that incorporates designated work hours will help train your brain to associate specific times with focused productivity.

In a world dominated by technology, it is crucial to leverage digital tools that promote productivity rather than hinder it. Utilize productivity apps and software that enable you to block distracting websites or limit your time spent on social media platforms. These tools can serve as virtual gatekeepers, allowing you to allocate your time and attention more effectively.

Another effective technique for minimizing distractions is practicing mindful work habits. Mindfulness involves being fully present and engaged in the task at hand, without being consumed by external thoughts or interruptions. By practicing mindfulness, you can train your mind to remain focused and avoid getting sidetracked.

Moreover, establishing clear boundaries with those around you is vital for maintaining productivity during the pandemic. Communicate your work schedule and expectations with family members or roommates to minimize interruptions and create a conducive work environment. Similarly, setting realistic goals and prioritizing tasks will help you stay on track and avoid feeling overwhelmed.

In conclusion, navigating the challenges of being productive during a pandemic requires a conscious effort to minimize distractions. By identifying and addressing potential distractions, creating a dedicated workspace, leveraging digital tools, practicing mindfulness, and setting boundaries, you can maximize your productivity levels and achieve a healthy work-life equilibrium. Remember, it is essential to adapt these strategies to suit your individual needs and circumstances. With perseverance and determination, you can thrive in this new normal and emerge stronger than ever.

Nurturing Relationships and Personal Connections

In this subchapter, we delve into the importance of nurturing relationships and personal connections, especially in the context of the ongoing pandemic. As we navigate through these uncertain times, it becomes increasingly crucial to prioritize our connections with others, both personally and professionally. Developing and maintaining these connections not only enhances our overall well-being but also contributes to our productivity and success during the pandemic.

The pandemic has forced us to adapt to new ways of living and working, with remote work becoming the norm for many. While this shift has brought certain benefits, such as increased flexibility and saved commuting time, it has also created a sense of isolation for many individuals. As humans, we thrive on social interactions, and the absence of face-to-face connections can have a significant impact on our mental health and productivity.

One way to counteract this isolation is by actively nurturing our relationships. This involves making a conscious effort to reach out to loved ones, friends, and colleagues. Whether it's through virtual hangouts, phone calls, or even sending a heartfelt message, these small gestures can go a long way in maintaining and strengthening our personal connections. By engaging in meaningful conversations and expressing our care and support, we not only uplift others but also cultivate a sense of belonging and purpose in our own lives.

Additionally, nurturing relationships can extend to professional connections as well. Despite the physical distance, it is crucial to stay connected with colleagues, clients, and mentors. Virtual meetings and collaborative platforms offer opportunities to foster teamwork, brainstorm ideas, and maintain professional networks. By actively engaging in these interactions, we can enhance our productivity, seek guidance, and establish a support system that aids in overcoming challenges during the pandemic.

Furthermore, nurturing relationships and personal connections can also involve self-reflection and self-care. Taking the time to understand our own needs and emotions allows us to communicate effectively with others and build healthier relationships. Engaging in activities that bring us joy, practicing mindfulness, and prioritizing self-care routines contribute to our overall well-being and resilience in the face of adversity.

In conclusion, nurturing relationships and personal connections is essential for everyone, particularly during the pandemic. By actively reaching out, engaging in meaningful conversations, and fostering connections both personally and professionally, we can combat the feelings of isolation and enhance our productivity. Remember, the power of connection lies within each of us, and by prioritizing relationships, we can achieve a harmonious work-life equilibrium for everyone.

Maintaining social connections while physically distant

In these unprecedented times, the COVID-19 pandemic has forced us to adapt to a new way of living. As we continue to practice social distancing, it is crucial to find alternative ways to maintain our social connections. Human beings are inherently social creatures, and our well-being depends on the relationships we nurture with others. This subchapter aims to provide you with some valuable insights and practical tips on how to stay connected with your loved ones, colleagues, and friends, even when physically distant.

1. Embrace Virtual Communication: With the advancement of technology, we are fortunate to have various platforms that facilitate virtual communication. Make the most of video conferencing tools like Zoom, Microsoft Teams, or Google Meet to connect with your family, friends, and colleagues. Schedule regular virtual meetups, happy hours, or game nights to recreate the sense of togetherness.

2. Prioritize Quality Time: In these challenging times, it is crucial to make time for your loved ones. Dedicate specific hours each week to connect with family and friends, focusing on quality interactions. Engage in meaningful conversations, share your experiences, and actively listen to others. This will strengthen your relationships and provide emotional support during these uncertain times.

3. Join Online Communities: Take advantage of online platforms and communities that cater to your interests and hobbies. Whether it's a virtual book club, cooking class, or fitness group, participating in such communities can help you connect with like-minded individuals who share similar passions. Engaging in common activities will not only

keep you socially connected but also enhance your productivity during the pandemic.

4. Show Empathy and Kindness: Remember that everyone is experiencing the pandemic differently, and some may be more isolated than others. Reach out to those who may be feeling lonely or struggling emotionally. Offer a listening ear, lend a helping hand, or simply check in on them regularly. Small acts of kindness go a long way in fostering social connections and supporting one another.

5. Rediscover Old Hobbies: Use this time to reconnect with yourself and rediscover old hobbies or develop new ones. Engaging in activities that bring you joy and fulfillment will not only make you more productive but also provide opportunities for social interaction. Join online classes, workshops, or virtual interest groups related to your hobbies to meet others who share your passion.

While physical distance may separate us, it does not have to diminish our social connections. By embracing virtual communication, prioritizing quality time, joining online communities, showing empathy, and rediscovering old hobbies, we can maintain strong social connections and achieve work-life equilibrium during this pandemic. Remember, we are all in this together, and by supporting one another, we can come out stronger and more connected than ever before.

Strengthening relationships with loved ones

In the midst of a pandemic, it is crucial to recognize the importance of nurturing and strengthening our relationships with loved ones. As we navigate the challenges of maintaining productivity during these uncertain times, it becomes even more vital to prioritize the connections that bring joy and support to our lives.

The pandemic has forced us into isolation, physically distancing ourselves from family and friends. However, this does not mean we have to distance ourselves emotionally. In fact, it presents an opportunity to explore creative ways to strengthen our relationships.

One way to achieve this is by embracing technology. With the advent of video conferencing platforms, we can now connect with our loved ones virtually, no matter the distance. Schedule regular virtual gatherings with family and friends, whether it be a weekly game night or a virtual dinner date. Engaging in these activities together will not only foster a sense of togetherness but also create lasting memories.

Another powerful tool to strengthen relationships is effective communication. During these trying times, it is crucial to be understanding and empathetic towards one another. Take the time to actively listen and engage in meaningful conversations. Share your thoughts, fears, and aspirations. By doing so, you create a safe space for open dialogue, allowing your loved ones to feel supported and valued.

Furthermore, it is important to remember that quality time does not necessarily mean physical presence. Engage in activities together, even if it is done remotely. Cook a meal together over video call, watch a movie simultaneously, or engage in a shared hobby. These shared experiences will help create a sense of connectedness and strengthen the bond between you and your loved ones.

Lastly, prioritize self-care. Taking care of your own physical and mental well-being is essential in maintaining healthy relationships. By ensuring you are in a good place mentally and emotionally, you will be better equipped to support and be present for your loved ones.

In conclusion, while the pandemic may have challenged our ability to be productive, it has also provided an opportunity to strengthen our relationships with loved ones. Embrace technology, communicate effectively, and engage in shared experiences to foster a sense of togetherness. By prioritizing these relationships, we can find balance and achieve work-life equilibrium, even in the midst of a pandemic.

Investing time in self-reflection and personal growth

In the midst of the global pandemic, life as we know it has been turned upside down. Our routines have been disrupted, our social interactions limited, and our work-life balance thrown completely off track. However, amidst the chaos and uncertainty, there lies an opportunity for personal growth and self-reflection. By investing time in ourselves during this challenging period, we can emerge stronger, more self-aware, and better equipped to achieve work-life equilibrium.

Self-reflection is an essential tool for personal growth. It allows us to examine our thoughts, behaviors, and emotions, and gain a deeper understanding of ourselves. During the pandemic, with fewer distractions and more time spent alone, we have a unique chance to engage in introspection. Take the time to ask yourself important questions: What truly matters to you? Are you satisfied with your current work-life balance? What areas of your life do you want to improve? By delving into these areas, you can unearth valuable insights that will guide you towards a more fulfilling and balanced life.

Investing time in personal growth is also crucial for being productive during the pandemic. As our work and personal lives blend together in the confines of our homes, it becomes increasingly challenging to maintain focus and motivation. Engaging in activities that promote personal growth, such as reading, learning a new skill, or practicing mindfulness, can help us stay grounded and motivated. These activities not only provide a sense of accomplishment but also contribute to our overall well-being, which is vital during these stressful times.

Furthermore, personal growth helps us adapt to the rapidly changing circumstances brought about by the pandemic. By developing new skills and expanding our knowledge base, we become more resilient and adaptable. This allows us to navigate the uncertainties of the current situation with greater ease and confidence. Moreover, personal growth fosters creativity and innovation, enabling us to find new solutions and opportunities amidst the challenges we face.

Ultimately, investing time in self-reflection and personal growth is an investment in ourselves. It is a commitment to our well-being, happiness, and success. By dedicating time each day to self-reflection and engaging in activities that promote personal growth, we can emerge from the pandemic with a renewed sense of purpose, a clearer vision of our goals, and the tools to achieve work-life equilibrium.

So, embrace this unique time and make the most of it. Invest in yourself, explore your passions, and discover new ways to grow. The pandemic may have disrupted our lives, but it has also given us an unprecedented opportunity for personal transformation. Seize it, and let it propel you towards a more balanced and fulfilling life.

Chapter 3: Overcoming Challenges and Adapting to Change

Overcoming Remote Work Challenges

In recent times, the COVID-19 pandemic has forced millions of individuals around the world to adapt to a new way of working – remote work. While this shift has undoubtedly brought about several advantages, such as flexibility and increased autonomy, it has also presented its fair share of challenges. In this subchapter, we will explore these obstacles and provide practical strategies to overcome them, ensuring that you can maintain productivity and achieve work-life equilibrium during these uncertain times.

One of the primary challenges of remote work is the blurring of boundaries between personal and professional life. When your home becomes your office, it can be difficult to establish a clear separation between work and leisure time. To overcome this, it is crucial to set and maintain a consistent schedule. Designate specific working hours and create a dedicated workspace that is separate from your living area. By doing so, you can create a psychological boundary that helps you switch into work mode and maintain focus during designated working hours.

Another common challenge faced by remote workers is the potential for isolation and feelings of loneliness. Without the social interactions that come naturally in a traditional office environment, it is essential to actively seek out opportunities for connection. Schedule regular virtual meetings or coffee breaks with colleagues, engage in online communities or forums related to your industry, and make an effort to stay connected with friends and family outside of work. Building a support network and maintaining social connections can help combat feelings of isolation and boost overall well-being.

Distractions and interruptions are also prevalent obstacles to productivity while working remotely. When your home becomes your office, it can be tempting to succumb to household chores, family demands, or the allure of social media. To overcome these distractions, establish clear boundaries with those around you, communicate your working hours, and create a daily routine that includes breaks to recharge and refocus. Additionally, utilizing productivity tools such as time-tracking apps or website blockers can help you stay on track and minimize distractions.

In conclusion, while remote work has its challenges, it is possible to overcome them and achieve work-life equilibrium during the pandemic. By setting boundaries, maintaining social connections, and implementing strategies to minimize distractions, you can enhance your productivity and well-being in the remote work environment. Embracing these strategies will not only benefit your work-life balance but also contribute to your overall satisfaction and success in these unprecedented times.

Managing isolation and loneliness

In times of crisis, such as the ongoing global pandemic, it is natural to feel a sense of isolation and loneliness. The sudden disruption to our daily lives, the physical distancing measures, and the lack of social gatherings have all contributed to a heightened feeling of disconnect. However, it is important to remember that we are all in this together, and there are ways to manage and overcome these feelings.

One of the key factors in managing isolation and loneliness is maintaining a sense of routine. With many of us now working from home, it is crucial to establish a daily schedule that includes regular breaks and time for social interaction. This could involve setting aside specific times for video calls with loved ones, participating in online communities, or even joining virtual hobby groups. By incorporating these activities into our routines, we can ensure that we are actively engaging with others and combating feelings of isolation.

Another effective strategy is to focus on self-care. During times of isolation, it is easy to neglect our own well-being. However, taking care of ourselves is essential for maintaining good mental health. This could involve engaging in activities that bring us joy, such as reading, exercising, or pursuing hobbies. Additionally, practicing mindfulness and meditation can help alleviate feelings of loneliness by grounding us in the present moment and fostering a sense of inner peace.

Furthermore, staying connected with our loved ones is vital. While physical gatherings may not be possible, we can make use of technology to bridge the gap. Regular video calls, phone conversations, or even sending letters can help maintain and strengthen our relationships. It is important to reach out to others and check in on their well-being as well. By supporting one another, we can combat the feelings of isolation and loneliness collectively.

Lastly, it is crucial to remember that we are not alone in this experience. The pandemic has affected people from all walks of life, and many are facing similar challenges. Seeking support from others who are going through similar situations can provide a sense of camaraderie and understanding. Online support groups and forums can offer a safe space to share experiences, seek advice, and find emotional support.

In conclusion, managing isolation and loneliness during the pandemic requires deliberate effort and self-care. By establishing routines, practicing self-care, staying connected with loved ones, and seeking support from others, we can combat these feelings and achieve a sense of equilibrium in our work-life dynamics. Remember, we are all in this together, and together we will overcome the pandemic paradox.

Overcoming technological barriers and connectivity issues

In today's interconnected world, technology has become an integral part of our lives. From smartphones to laptops, we rely on these devices to stay connected and productive, especially during the ongoing pandemic. However, as convenient as technology may be, it also presents its fair share of challenges. This subchapter aims to explore the various technological barriers and connectivity issues that individuals face during these testing times, and provides practical solutions to overcome them.

One of the most common obstacles faced by many individuals is the lack of access to reliable internet connectivity. Whether due to living in remote areas or financial constraints, not everyone has high-speed internet at their disposal. This can hinder productivity and leave individuals feeling disconnected. To overcome this barrier, several options can be explored, such as utilizing public Wi-Fi hotspots, collaborating with neighbors for shared internet, or seeking assistance from local community organizations that provide internet access.

Another challenge that arises is the struggle to adapt to new technologies and digital tools. The rapid advancement of technology can leave some individuals feeling overwhelmed and unsure of how to navigate the ever-evolving digital landscape. To address this barrier, it is crucial to invest in digital literacy programs that educate individuals on the basics of using technology effectively. Online tutorials, webinars, and workshops can provide valuable guidance and empower individuals to become more tech-savvy, thus enhancing their productivity during the pandemic.

Moreover, it is essential to recognize the issue of technological inequality that exists among different socioeconomic groups. Not everyone has equal access to the latest gadgets or the resources to upgrade their devices. To bridge this gap, governments, organizations, and individuals can come together to provide refurbished laptops or tablets to those in need. Additionally, companies can offer subsidies or discounts on internet plans to make it more affordable for everyone.

In conclusion, overcoming technological barriers and connectivity issues is crucial for individuals to remain productive during the pandemic. By addressing the lack of reliable internet access, providing digital literacy programs, and reducing technological inequality, we can ensure that everyone has the opportunity to thrive in a digital world. It is through these collective efforts that we can achieve work-life equilibrium for everyone, enabling individuals to navigate the challenges of the pandemic while staying connected and productive.

Building a virtual support network

In the midst of the global pandemic, many of us have found ourselves in uncharted territory, navigating the challenges of working from home while trying to maintain a sense of normalcy in our lives. Suddenly, we are faced with the need to be productive during a time of uncertainty and isolation. It is in these moments that building a virtual support network becomes crucial.

A virtual support network can be defined as a group of individuals who provide emotional, professional, and social support, all through digital means. In the absence of physical interactions, these networks have become a lifeline for many, helping to combat feelings of loneliness and fostering a sense of belonging.

One of the first steps in building a virtual support network is identifying your needs and interests. Are you seeking professional guidance, emotional support, or simply a sense of community? Once you have identified your needs, you can begin to reach out to others who share similar interests or goals.

There are various platforms available that can help facilitate this process. Social media groups, online forums, and professional networking sites are all excellent resources for connecting with like-minded individuals. Joining these communities allows you to engage in discussions, seek advice, and share experiences with others who are facing similar challenges.

In addition to joining existing communities, consider creating your own virtual support network. Reach out to friends, colleagues, or acquaintances who you believe would benefit from such a network.

Utilize video conferencing tools to schedule regular meetings or virtual coffee chats, where you can discuss your struggles, share tips for productivity, and provide support to one another.

Remember, building a virtual support network is not just about receiving support, but also about giving it. Actively engage with others, offer assistance and encouragement, and be a source of inspiration for those who may be struggling. By contributing to the network, you create a positive and uplifting environment for everyone involved.

In conclusion, building a virtual support network is essential for maintaining productivity during the pandemic. It provides a sense of community, emotional support, and professional guidance, all of which are crucial for achieving a work-life equilibrium. Whether you join existing communities or create your own, nurturing these connections will not only benefit you but also contribute to the well-being of others. Embrace the power of virtual support networks and discover the strength in unity during these challenging times.

Embracing Flexibility and Resilience

In the midst of the global pandemic, our lives have been upended, and the boundaries between work and personal life have become blurred like never before. The challenges of balancing work responsibilities with personal well-being have become more apparent, making the need to embrace flexibility and resilience crucial in achieving a harmonious work-life equilibrium.

For everyone, the pandemic has brought about a unique set of circumstances that require us to adapt and find new ways to be productive. Whether you are a parent juggling remote work and homeschooling, an essential worker facing increased demands and risks, or someone grappling with the uncertainties of job security, finding the right balance is essential for both mental and physical well-being.

Flexibility is the key to navigating these uncharted waters. It requires us to reimagine the traditional notions of work and productivity. Embracing flexibility means acknowledging that each day may bring different challenges and finding creative solutions to overcome them. It may involve adjusting work hours to accommodate personal obligations, setting realistic goals, and focusing on the tasks that truly matter. By prioritizing flexibility, we can reduce stress and enhance our ability to adapt to changing circumstances.

Resilience is equally important in this journey towards work-life equilibrium. It serves as a foundation for navigating the uncertainties and setbacks that the pandemic has brought upon us. Resilience allows us to bounce back from challenges, learn from failures, and cultivate a positive mindset. It involves developing coping mechanisms, seeking support from loved ones, and building a strong support network. By embracing resilience, we can maintain our productivity and mental well-being in the face of adversity.

For those seeking to be productive during the pandemic, it is essential to remember that productivity is not solely measured by the number of tasks completed or hours worked. It is about finding a balance that allows you to meet your professional obligations while also taking care of yourself and your loved ones. By embracing flexibility and resilience, you can create a work-life equilibrium that promotes both productivity and personal well-being.

In conclusion, the pandemic has presented us with unprecedented challenges, but it has also given us an opportunity to redefine work-life equilibrium. By embracing flexibility and resilience, we can navigate these uncertain times with grace and achieve a harmonious balance between work and personal life. Remember, it is not about striving for perfection but rather finding a balance that works for you and allows you to thrive in these trying times.

Adapting to changing work demands and expectations

In the midst of a global pandemic, the way we work has undergone drastic transformations. As we navigate through uncertain times, it becomes essential to understand how to adapt to changing work demands and expectations. This subchapter explores strategies and insights to help individuals be productive during the pandemic while maintaining a healthy work-life equilibrium.

The pandemic has brought about a shift in the traditional work environment, with remote work becoming the new norm for many. As individuals find themselves adjusting to this new reality, it is crucial to establish a structured routine that balances work and personal life. Setting clear boundaries between the two domains ensures that work does not encroach upon personal time and vice versa. Creating a designated workspace within your home can also enhance focus and productivity.

Moreover, the pandemic has accelerated the need for flexibility and agility in the workplace. Adapting to changing demands requires individuals to develop new skills and stay up-to-date with the latest industry trends. Embracing online learning platforms and seeking out professional development opportunities can help individuals stay ahead in their careers. Additionally, fostering a growth mindset and being open to change can enable individuals to adapt more effectively to new work expectations.

The pandemic has also highlighted the importance of mental well-being in maintaining productivity. Taking care of one's mental health has become paramount during these challenging times. Prioritizing self-care activities such as exercise, meditation, and maintaining social connections can help reduce stress and increase resilience. Employers can play a vital role in supporting their employees' well-being by providing resources for mental health support and promoting a healthy work-life balance.

Furthermore, effective communication and collaboration have become crucial in the remote work landscape. Employing digital tools for virtual meetings, project management, and team collaboration can facilitate seamless communication and enhance productivity. Regular check-ins with colleagues and managers can help alleviate feelings of isolation and ensure a sense of belonging within the team.

In conclusion, adapting to changing work demands and expectations during the pandemic requires individuals to establish a structured routine, develop new skills, prioritize mental well-being, and embrace effective communication and collaboration. By implementing these strategies, individuals can navigate the challenges of remote work while maintaining a healthy work-life equilibrium. The pandemic may have disrupted our lives, but it also presents an opportunity to embrace change and find innovative ways to thrive in the new work landscape.

Embracing a growth mindset and embracing opportunities for learning

In the midst of a global pandemic, it is easy to feel overwhelmed, uncertain, and even stagnant in our personal and professional lives. However, it is during these challenging times that embracing a growth mindset becomes even more crucial. In this subchapter, we will explore how cultivating a growth mindset can help individuals be productive during the pandemic and seize unique opportunities for learning and personal development.

A growth mindset is the belief that abilities, talents, and intelligence can be developed through dedication, effort, and a willingness to learn. By adopting this mindset, individuals can embrace challenges, persist in the face of setbacks, and see failure as an opportunity for growth rather than a limitation. This perspective becomes especially relevant when navigating through a pandemic, where adaptability and resilience are essential.

Being productive during a pandemic requires a shift in mindset. Instead of focusing solely on the obstacles and limitations imposed by the crisis, individuals should seek out opportunities for growth and learning. This can be achieved by setting achievable goals, developing new skills, and seeking out learning experiences that align with personal or professional interests. By adopting a growth mindset, individuals can turn a crisis into an opportunity for personal and professional development.

The pandemic has forced individuals to adapt to new ways of working and living. Remote work, virtual meetings, and online learning have become the norm. Embracing these changes and exploring innovative ways to be productive can lead to new opportunities and skill development. It is crucial to embrace technology, explore new tools and platforms, and seek out professional development resources to adapt and thrive in this new environment.

Moreover, a growth mindset allows individuals to view setbacks and challenges as learning opportunities. Instead of being discouraged by failures or setbacks, individuals can examine them objectively, learn from them, and adjust their approach. This mindset fosters resilience, adaptability, and a continuous drive for improvement.

In conclusion, embracing a growth mindset and seizing opportunities for learning are critical to being productive during the pandemic. By adopting a growth mindset, individuals can overcome challenges, adapt to new circumstances, and see setbacks as opportunities for growth. This mindset shift allows for personal and professional development, leading to a more fulfilling and successful life, even in the face of adversity.

Resilience-building practices to cope with uncertainty

In these unprecedented times, the COVID-19 pandemic has brought about a wave of uncertainty that has affected individuals from all walks of life. The sudden shift in our work and personal lives has left many feeling overwhelmed and uncertain about the future. However, it is during times like these that building resilience becomes essential to maintain a sense of balance and cope with uncertainty effectively.

Resilience is the ability to bounce back from adversity and adapt to change. It is a quality that can be cultivated through various practices, helping us navigate through difficult times and emerge stronger on the other side. In this subchapter, we will explore some resilience-building practices that can empower individuals to stay productive during the pandemic and achieve work-life equilibrium.

First and foremost, maintaining a positive mindset is crucial. It is natural to feel anxious or overwhelmed, but focusing on the positives can help shift our perspective. Practicing gratitude daily, by acknowledging and appreciating the things we have, can foster a sense of resilience and optimism.

Another important practice is establishing a routine. With the blurring of boundaries between work and personal life, it is imperative to create a structured schedule that allows for balance and productivity. Setting clear boundaries, both in terms of time and physical space, can help create a sense of stability and enable individuals to switch off from work when needed.

Additionally, nurturing social connections, albeit virtually, is vital during these times of isolation. Engaging in regular check-ins with friends, family, and colleagues can provide support and a sense of belonging. Collaborating and sharing experiences with others facing similar challenges can foster a collective resilience that is invaluable.

Furthermore, taking care of physical and mental well-being is crucial for resilience-building. Engaging in regular exercise, practicing mindfulness or meditation, and ensuring adequate sleep are all essential components of self-care. These practices not only boost our immune system but also enhance our mental and emotional well-being, equipping us to handle uncertainty more effectively.

Lastly, embracing adaptability is key. The pandemic has forced us to adapt to new ways of working and living. Cultivating a growth mindset and being open to change can help us navigate uncertainty with ease. Embracing new technologies, learning new skills, and being flexible in our approach are all integral aspects of building resilience.

In conclusion, the COVID-19 pandemic has presented us with numerous challenges, but it is through resilience-building practices that we can navigate these uncertain times successfully. By cultivating a positive mindset, establishing routines, nurturing social connections, prioritizing well-being, and embracing adaptability, we can achieve work-life equilibrium and remain productive despite the pandemic's challenges. Remember, resilience is not something we are born with; it is a skill that can be developed and honed with practice.

Chapter 4: Creating a Culture of Work-Life Equilibrium

Employer Responsibility: Fostering Work-Life Balance

In the midst of the ongoing pandemic, individuals around the world are facing unprecedented challenges in maintaining a healthy work-life balance. The boundaries between work and personal life have become blurred, leading to increased stress, burnout, and decreased productivity. It is crucial for employers to recognize their responsibility in fostering work-life balance for their employees, not only for the well-being of their workforce but also for the success of their organizations.

The first step in promoting work-life balance is understanding its significance. Work-life balance refers to the equilibrium between professional responsibilities and personal well-being. It is a state in which individuals can effectively manage their workloads while still having time for family, hobbies, and self-care. By achieving this balance, employees are more likely to be engaged, motivated, and productive.

Employers can play a pivotal role in creating a work environment that supports work-life balance. This can be done by implementing flexible work arrangements, such as remote work options or flexible scheduling. By allowing employees to have control over their work hours and location, employers empower them to better manage their personal responsibilities, such as caring for children or elderly parents, while still meeting work obligations.

Additionally, employers should encourage regular breaks and discourage overworking. Burnout has become a significant concern during the pandemic, as the boundaries between work and personal life have become blurred. By promoting the importance of taking breaks and setting clear expectations for work hours, employers can help prevent burnout and promote overall well-being.

Another crucial aspect of fostering work-life balance is promoting open communication and creating a supportive work culture. Employers should ensure that employees feel comfortable discussing their work-life balance needs and concerns. This can be achieved through regular check-ins, employee surveys, or even designated support groups. By actively listening to employees' needs, employers can implement necessary changes and provide the resources and support required to maintain work-life equilibrium.

Ultimately, fostering work-life balance is a win-win situation for both employees and employers. Employees who are able to achieve a healthy work-life balance are more likely to be satisfied, motivated, and committed to their jobs. In turn, this translates into increased productivity, reduced turnover rates, and improved organizational performance.

In conclusion, the responsibility to foster work-life balance lies with employers, especially during the pandemic. By implementing flexible work arrangements, discouraging overworking, promoting open communication, and creating a supportive work culture, employers can empower their employees to achieve work-life equilibrium. In doing so, they not only enhance the well-being of their workforce but also create a more productive and successful organization.

Implementing flexible work policies and practices

In the wake of the global COVID-19 pandemic, the world witnessed a massive shift in the way we work. As organizations scrambled to adapt to the new normal, the concept of flexible work policies and practices emerged as a crucial solution to maintain productivity, employee well-being, and work-life equilibrium. This subchapter explores the importance of implementing flexible work policies and practices and how they can benefit everyone, especially those seeking to be productive during the pandemic.

Flexibility in work arrangements has become a necessity in the face of the pandemic. Companies that successfully implemented flexible work policies saw increased employee satisfaction and engagement, leading to higher productivity levels. By allowing employees to work remotely or providing flexible hours, organizations have enabled individuals to balance their personal and professional responsibilities effectively. This flexibility has been particularly valuable for individuals with caregiving responsibilities, allowing them to manage their work and family commitments simultaneously.

Moreover, flexible work policies have proven to be a great equalizer, providing opportunities for people from diverse backgrounds to thrive. Remote work has eliminated geographical limitations, opening doors for individuals who were previously hindered by location-based restrictions. This inclusivity has resulted in a more diverse and dynamic workforce, fostering an environment that embraces new ideas and perspectives.

Implementing flexible work policies and practices requires a strategic approach. Organizations must consider factors such as job roles, technological infrastructure, and employee preferences. Communication and collaboration tools, along with supportive management practices, are vital to ensure seamless remote work. Regular check-ins, virtual team-building activities, and transparent goal-setting can help maintain a sense of connection and motivation among employees.

However, it is important to acknowledge that flexible work is not a one-size-fits-all solution. Some individuals thrive in a remote work environment, while others may struggle with isolation or find it challenging to separate work and personal life. Organizations must prioritize individual needs and provide support accordingly, offering resources for mental health and work-life balance.

In conclusion, implementing flexible work policies and practices is crucial in achieving work-life equilibrium for everyone during the pandemic. This approach enhances productivity, promotes employee well-being, and fosters a diverse and inclusive work environment. By embracing flexibility, organizations can adapt to the evolving work landscape and ensure that individuals can thrive both personally and professionally.

Promoting employee well-being and mental health support

In these unprecedented times of the pandemic, it has become more crucial than ever to prioritize employee well-being and mental health support. As the world grapples with the challenges of remote work, social isolation, and uncertainty, organizations must take proactive steps to ensure the well-being of their employees. In this subchapter, we will explore strategies for promoting employee well-being and providing essential mental health support during these challenging times.

One of the most effective ways to support employees' well-being is by fostering a positive work environment. Encouraging open communication, empathy, and understanding among team members can significantly contribute to their overall mental health. Regular check-ins, virtual team-building activities, and creating opportunities for social interaction can help combat feelings of isolation and promote a sense of belonging.

Organizations should also prioritize providing resources and tools for managing stress and maintaining work-life equilibrium. This may include offering virtual wellness programs, mindfulness sessions, or providing access to mental health professionals through employee assistance programs. By acknowledging the unique challenges employees face during the pandemic and offering tailored support, organizations can help alleviate stress and promote a healthier work-life balance.

Furthermore, leaders should lead by example and encourage self-care practices among their teams. Taking breaks, setting boundaries, and promoting a healthy work-life integration can help employees maintain their productivity and overall well-being. Additionally, fostering a culture that values work-life equilibrium rather than overwork or burnout can have a positive impact on both individuals and the organization as a whole.

In conclusion, promoting employee well-being and mental health support is essential in maintaining productivity during the pandemic. By creating a supportive work environment, providing resources for stress management, and promoting self-care practices, organizations can foster a healthier and more productive workforce. It is crucial for organizations to recognize the challenges faced by employees and take proactive measures to address their mental health needs. By doing so, we can navigate through the pandemic paradox and achieve work-life equilibrium for everyone.

Encouraging work-life integration rather than separation

In the face of the ongoing pandemic, our lives have been dramatically altered. The lines between work and personal life have become increasingly blurry, with many of us finding ourselves working from the comfort of our homes. While this new reality may initially seem daunting, it also presents a unique opportunity to embrace work-life integration rather than separation.

Traditionally, the idea of work-life balance has been emphasized, with the belief that the two should be kept separate to ensure personal well-being. However, in our current circumstances, this approach may no longer be feasible or even desirable. Instead, we can strive to achieve work-life integration, where the boundaries between work and personal life are more fluid and flexible.

Embracing work-life integration allows us to find harmony in our daily lives, enabling us to be more productive during this challenging time. By integrating work and personal responsibilities, we can create a schedule that accommodates both, leading to increased efficiency and reduced stress. This approach also enables us to be present for our loved ones, fostering stronger relationships and overall well-being.

To encourage work-life integration, it is crucial to establish clear boundaries and routines. Start by designating specific workspaces in your home, separate from areas dedicated to relaxation and personal activities. This physical separation can help create a mental distinction between work and personal life, allowing you to switch between the two more effectively.

Additionally, setting realistic goals and priorities can prevent feelings of overwhelm and ensure that both work and personal tasks are given the attention they deserve. Take breaks throughout the day to recharge and engage in activities that bring you joy. This could include spending quality time with your family, pursuing hobbies, or simply taking a walk in nature.

Moreover, open communication and collaboration with colleagues and family members are essential. Clearly communicate your availability and establish boundaries with your colleagues, ensuring that they respect your personal time. By involving your loved ones in your work-life integration journey, you can gain their support and understanding.

The pandemic has forced us to reevaluate our approach to work and personal life. By embracing work-life integration, we can find a sense of equilibrium during these challenging times. Remember, it is not about achieving a perfect balance, but rather about finding harmony and fulfillment in both aspects of our lives. Together, we can navigate the pandemic paradox and emerge stronger, more resilient, and truly productive.

The Importance of Self-Advocacy in Achieving Equilibrium

In the midst of the global pandemic, achieving work-life equilibrium seems like an elusive goal for many. The constant juggling of work responsibilities, household chores, and personal well-being can easily lead to burnout and a sense of imbalance. However, there is a powerful tool that can help individuals navigate these challenging times and find a harmonious balance – self-advocacy.

Self-advocacy is the ability to speak up for oneself, assert personal needs, and actively seek support and resources. It is a crucial skill that empowers individuals to take control of their own lives and create a sense of equilibrium in the face of uncertainty. During these unprecedented times, self-advocacy becomes even more important in ensuring productivity and maintaining overall well-being.

One of the key aspects of self-advocacy is setting boundaries. As individuals continue to work from home and face the blurring of lines between professional and personal life, it is essential to establish clear boundaries to maintain productivity. This could mean setting specific working hours, designating a separate workspace, or communicating expectations with colleagues and family members. By advocating for these boundaries, individuals can create a conducive environment for work while also nurturing personal relationships and self-care.

Self-advocacy also involves recognizing and addressing personal needs. The pandemic has brought about unique challenges, such as increased stress, isolation, and mental health issues. By advocating for oneself, individuals can seek out the necessary support systems, such as therapy, online communities, or wellness resources. Taking the initiative to prioritize mental and emotional well-being is essential in maintaining productivity and achieving equilibrium in all aspects of life.

Furthermore, self-advocacy extends beyond personal needs and encompasses professional growth as well. In a time where career advancement may seem uncertain, individuals can advocate for themselves by seeking out professional development opportunities, networking virtually, or taking on new projects. By actively advocating for their skills and goals, individuals can continue to grow and thrive in their careers, even during the pandemic.

In conclusion, self-advocacy plays a vital role in achieving work-life equilibrium during these challenging times. By setting boundaries, recognizing personal needs, and advocating for professional growth, individuals can navigate the complexities of the pandemic with resilience and balance. It is essential for everyone to embrace the power of self-advocacy and prioritize their well-being in order to achieve a sense of equilibrium amidst the pandemic paradox.

Communicating personal needs and boundaries effectively

In the midst of the ongoing pandemic, finding a balance between work and personal life has become more challenging than ever. As we navigate through these uncertain times, it is crucial to prioritize our mental and emotional well-being by effectively communicating our personal needs and setting boundaries. By doing so, we can maintain productivity, while also nurturing our overall happiness and fulfillment.

Communication is the key to building strong relationships, both personally and professionally. When it comes to expressing our needs and setting boundaries, clear and open communication becomes even more essential. It is important to remember that everyone's situation is unique, and what works for one person may not work for another. By effectively communicating our personal needs, we can ensure that others understand our limitations, preferences, and concerns.

One effective way to communicate our needs is by setting clear boundaries. Boundaries act as guidelines that define the limits of what is acceptable to us. During the pandemic, it is essential to set boundaries between work and personal life, as many of us are now working remotely. Establishing specific working hours can help maintain a healthy work-life balance, allowing sufficient time for relaxation, family, and self-care. Communicate these boundaries clearly with your employer, colleagues, and loved ones, and kindly ask for their cooperation in respecting your personal space and time.

Additionally, effective communication involves active listening. When someone shares their personal needs or boundaries with us, it is important to listen attentively and validate their concerns. By showing empathy and understanding, we can foster an environment of trust and respect. This reciprocity can encourage others to reciprocate the same level of understanding, making it easier for everyone to communicate their needs openly.

In conclusion, effectively communicating personal needs and boundaries is crucial for achieving work-life equilibrium during the pandemic. By setting clear boundaries and openly expressing our limitations and concerns, we can maintain productivity while nurturing our overall well-being. Remember, effective communication is a two-way street, so it is equally important to actively listen and validate the needs of others. Let us strive to create a supportive and empathetic environment where everyone's personal needs and boundaries are respected for the benefit of all.

Negotiating work arrangements and accommodations

In today's ever-changing work landscape, the COVID-19 pandemic has undoubtedly disrupted our traditional ways of working. As we strive to find a balance between work and life amidst these challenging times, negotiating work arrangements and accommodations has become increasingly crucial. This subchapter of "The Pandemic Paradox: Achieving Work-Life Equilibrium for Everyone" aims to guide you through the process of negotiating and implementing effective work arrangements that promote productivity and well-being during the pandemic.

First and foremost, it is essential to recognize that the pandemic has brought about a need for flexibility and adaptability in our work lives. Whether you are working remotely or on-site, negotiating with your employer or colleagues is key to establishing a conducive work environment. Open communication is vital in expressing your needs, concerns, and aspirations. By initiating a dialogue, you can explore various options that cater to both your personal and professional requirements.

Remote work has become an integral part of our lives, allowing us to maintain productivity while staying safe. However, it is essential to negotiate clear boundaries and expectations with your employer or team. Establishing a designated workspace, setting specific working hours, and defining deliverables can help create a structured routine and prevent work from encroaching upon personal time.

Moreover, negotiating accommodations for individuals with unique circumstances is critical to ensuring inclusivity during the pandemic.

Whether you are a parent juggling childcare responsibilities, a caregiver for a family member, or an individual with health concerns, discussing and implementing accommodations can alleviate stress and support your overall well-being. Flexibility in work hours, reduced workload, or modified tasks are potential accommodations that can be negotiated to meet your specific needs.

Remember, negotiation is a two-way street. While advocating for your needs, it is also essential to consider the interests of your employer or team. Highlighting the benefits of your proposed arrangements, such as increased productivity, reduced stress levels, or improved work-life balance, can help create a win-win situation for both parties involved.

In conclusion, negotiating work arrangements and accommodations is crucial for everyone striving to be productive during the pandemic. By engaging in open communication, establishing clear boundaries, and considering the interests of all parties, you can create a work environment that promotes well-being, productivity, and work-life equilibrium for all. Adaptability, flexibility, and empathy are the keys to navigating these challenging times successfully.

Empowering individuals to prioritize their well-being

In today's fast-paced world, the concept of work-life equilibrium has become increasingly elusive. However, the ongoing COVID-19 pandemic has forced us to reassess our priorities and seek a new balance between our personal and professional lives. In this subchapter titled "Empowering individuals to prioritize their well-being," we will explore strategies and insights to help you navigate the challenges of being productive during the pandemic while maintaining your overall well-being.

The pandemic has undoubtedly disrupted our routines and created a sense of uncertainty. As a result, it is crucial to prioritize our mental and physical health. One effective strategy is to establish a daily self-care routine that includes activities such as mindfulness exercises, regular exercise, and sufficient sleep. By dedicating time to take care of ourselves, we can enhance our overall well-being and increase our productivity in the long run.

Additionally, it is essential to set clear boundaries between work and personal life. Working from home has blurred the lines between these two domains, making it challenging to disconnect and recharge. Establishing a designated workspace and sticking to a schedule can help create a sense of structure and ensure that you have time for both work and personal activities. Remember, a healthy work-life balance is essential for your mental health and productivity.

Furthermore, empower yourself by embracing technology and seeking out virtual resources that can support your well-being. Online platforms offer a plethora of options, including virtual fitness classes, meditation apps, and counseling services. These resources can help you stay connected, maintain a healthy lifestyle, and seek support when needed.

Lastly, it is crucial to communicate openly with your employer or colleagues about your needs and limitations. Expressing your concerns and setting realistic expectations can lead to a more understanding and supportive work environment. Remember, you are not alone in facing the challenges of the pandemic, and by working together, we can all achieve work-life equilibrium.

In conclusion, prioritizing your well-being during the pandemic is crucial to maintaining productivity and achieving a healthy work-life balance. By establishing a self-care routine, setting boundaries, utilizing virtual resources, and fostering open communication, you can empower yourself to navigate these challenging times. Remember that your well-being is essential, and by taking care of yourself, you are better equipped to handle the demands of work and life. Let us embrace this opportunity to create a new equilibrium that prioritizes our overall well-being, as we navigate the pandemic together.

Chapter 5: Thriving in the New Normal: Sustaining Work-Life Equilibrium

Embracing a Hybrid Work Model

In the wake of the COVID-19 pandemic, the traditional work landscape has undergone a seismic shift. As organizations and individuals adapt to the new normal, one concept that has gained considerable traction is the hybrid work model. This subchapter explores the benefits and challenges of embracing this flexible approach and provides key insights on how to be productive during these uncertain times.

The hybrid work model combines the best of both worlds - the flexibility of remote work and the collaborative environment of the office. It allows employees to have the freedom to work remotely while still maintaining face-to-face interactions with colleagues when necessary. This newfound flexibility has proven to be a game-changer in achieving work-life equilibrium.

One of the primary advantages of the hybrid work model is increased productivity. Research shows that employees who have the autonomy to choose their work environment are more engaged and motivated. By eliminating lengthy commutes and providing a comfortable workspace, individuals can focus on their tasks without the distractions commonly found in a traditional office setting. Furthermore, the flexibility to manage personal commitments alongside work responsibilities leads to a healthier work-life balance, ultimately enhancing overall productivity and job satisfaction.

However, embracing a hybrid work model is not without its challenges. Effective communication and collaboration become crucial in this arrangement. Organizations must invest in robust technology solutions to facilitate seamless virtual meetings and project management. Clear communication channels and protocols should be established to ensure everyone is on the same page, regardless of their physical location. Additionally, managers need to adopt a results-oriented approach, shifting the focus from monitoring hours spent at the office to measuring outcomes and deliverables.

For individuals seeking to be productive during the pandemic, it is essential to establish a routine and create a dedicated workspace at home. Setting clear boundaries between work and personal life, such as implementing regular breaks and adhering to regular working hours, helps maintain focus and avoid burnout. Prioritizing tasks, leveraging technology tools for organization and time management, and practicing self-care are also key components of successfully navigating this hybrid work model.

In conclusion, embracing a hybrid work model offers numerous benefits for both organizations and individuals. By leveraging the flexibility of remote work while fostering collaboration in office settings, this model creates a conducive environment for productivity and work-life equilibrium. However, it requires effective communication, technology integration, and a results-oriented approach. By implementing these strategies, individuals can navigate the challenges of the pandemic and maintain their productivity, ultimately achieving a healthier work-life balance.

Balancing remote and in-person work arrangements

In the midst of the ongoing pandemic, the workplace landscape has undergone a significant transformation. With the rise of remote work, many individuals have found themselves navigating the challenges of finding a balance between working from home and returning to in-person work arrangements. This subchapter aims to provide guidance and insights on how to strike a harmonious equilibrium between these two modes of work, ensuring productivity and well-being in the process.

One of the key factors in successfully balancing remote and in-person work arrangements is effective time management. It is crucial to establish clear boundaries and allocate specific time slots for both remote and in-person work. This helps in maintaining a routine and ensuring that neither aspect of work overshadows the other. By setting aside dedicated hours for each mode, individuals can maximize their productivity and minimize distractions.

Another essential aspect is creating a conducive work environment, regardless of the location. When working remotely, it is crucial to designate a dedicated workspace that is free from distractions. This helps in maintaining focus and separating personal life from professional responsibilities. Similarly, when returning to in-person work, it is important to ensure a safe and comfortable environment that promotes collaboration and engagement.

Communication plays a pivotal role in balancing remote and in-person work arrangements. Regular and effective communication with colleagues, supervisors, and team members is crucial to stay connected and aligned. Leveraging technology tools such as video conferences, instant messaging, and project management platforms can bridge the gap between remote and in-person team members. By fostering open and transparent communication channels, individuals can maintain a sense of belonging and collaborative spirit, irrespective of their work arrangement.

Maintaining work-life harmony is another crucial aspect of balancing remote and in-person work arrangements. The flexibility that remote work offers can be leveraged to prioritize personal well-being and family responsibilities. However, it is equally important to establish boundaries and avoid overworking. By setting clear expectations and creating a healthy work-life balance, individuals can ensure that their productivity and overall well-being are not compromised.

In conclusion, balancing remote and in-person work arrangements is a delicate task that requires effective time management, a conducive work environment, open communication, and a focus on work-life harmony. By implementing these strategies, individuals can navigate the challenges of the pandemic and achieve work-life equilibrium. Whether working remotely or returning to in-person work, it is essential to prioritize productivity, well-being, and personal fulfillment.

Leveraging technology for efficient collaboration

In this rapidly evolving digital age, technology has become an indispensable tool for individuals and organizations alike. The ongoing pandemic has further accentuated the significance of technology, especially when it comes to collaborating and remaining productive in the face of adversity. In this subchapter, we will explore how we can harness the power of technology to enhance collaboration and achieve work-life equilibrium during these challenging times.

One of the most transformative aspects of technology is its ability to connect people from all corners of the world. Through virtual meetings, video conferencing, and collaboration platforms, individuals can seamlessly communicate and collaborate with their colleagues, irrespective of physical distance. This has proven to be a game-changer during the pandemic, enabling teams to continue their work remotely and maintain productivity levels.

The key to efficient collaboration lies in choosing the right tools and platforms that suit the unique needs of your team. There is a plethora of options available, ranging from communication applications like Slack and Microsoft Teams to project management tools like Trello and Asana. By leveraging these technologies, you can streamline workflows, assign tasks, monitor progress, and ensure everyone remains on the same page.

Moreover, the pandemic has also accelerated the adoption of cloud-based storage solutions. Cloud storage not only provides secure and centralized access to files but also allows for real-time collaboration on shared documents. This eliminates the need for multiple versions of files and reduces confusion, enabling seamless collaboration among team members.

Another aspect worth mentioning is the rise of virtual whiteboarding and brainstorming tools. These platforms enable teams to brainstorm ideas, share concepts, and collaborate in real-time, just as they would in a physical setting. By leveraging these tools, creative thinking can thrive, and innovation can continue to flourish despite the challenges posed by the pandemic.

Lastly, it is essential to acknowledge the importance of striking a balance between work and personal life during these times. Technology can be both a boon and a bane, as it blurs the boundaries between work and personal time. It is crucial to set clear boundaries and establish designated workspaces to maintain a healthy work-life equilibrium. Scheduling breaks, engaging in physical activities, and fostering open communication with colleagues can also contribute to overall well-being and productivity.

In conclusion, technology has emerged as a lifeline during the pandemic, enabling efficient collaboration and productivity. By leveraging the right tools and adopting best practices, individuals and organizations can navigate these challenging times while achieving a healthy work-life equilibrium. Embrace the power of technology, and unlock its potential to transform the way we work and collaborate, ensuring that productivity is not compromised, even during a global crisis.

Reaping the benefits of a flexible work environment

In today's rapidly changing world, the concept of a traditional 9-to-5 work environment has become increasingly outdated. The COVID-19 pandemic has forced many organizations to adapt and embrace a flexible work arrangement, and it's becoming evident that this shift offers numerous benefits for both employees and employers.

One of the primary advantages of a flexible work environment is the ability to achieve a better work-life balance. During the pandemic, many individuals have found themselves juggling multiple responsibilities, such as caring for children, managing household chores, and ensuring their own well-being. With a flexible work arrangement, individuals have the freedom to determine when and where they work, enabling them to better integrate their personal and professional lives. This newfound flexibility allows for increased productivity, reduced stress levels, and ultimately, a higher quality of life.

Moreover, a flexible work environment promotes employee satisfaction and engagement. When individuals have the autonomy to create their own work schedule and choose their preferred work setting, they feel a greater sense of control and ownership over their work. This, in turn, leads to increased motivation and a stronger commitment to achieving organizational goals. Employees who feel empowered and trusted by their employers are more likely to go above and beyond their job requirements, resulting in higher levels of productivity and creativity.

Additionally, a flexible work environment can have a positive impact on an organization's bottom line. By embracing remote work or flexible hours, employers can significantly reduce overhead costs associated with maintaining physical office spaces. This includes expenses related to rent, utilities, and office supplies. Furthermore, companies that offer flexible work arrangements often have a wider talent pool to choose from, as location is no longer a limiting factor. This allows organizations to attract and retain top talent from around the world, resulting in a diverse and highly skilled workforce.

As we navigate the challenges imposed by the pandemic, it's crucial to recognize the potential benefits of a flexible work environment. Whether you're a working professional, a parent, or someone seeking a better work-life equilibrium, embracing flexibility can be transformative. By reevaluating traditional work structures and embracing new ways of working, individuals and organizations can not only survive but thrive in the face of adversity.

In conclusion, the COVID-19 pandemic has accelerated the need for a flexible work environment. It offers numerous benefits, including a better work-life balance, increased employee satisfaction and engagement, and cost savings for organizations. By embracing flexibility, individuals and organizations can navigate the challenges posed by the pandemic and achieve a harmonious work-life equilibrium. It's time to seize the opportunity and reap the benefits of a flexible work environment.

The Future of Work-Life Equilibrium

In the midst of the global pandemic, the concept of work-life equilibrium has taken on a whole new meaning. As we navigate through these uncertain times, it has become increasingly important to strike a balance between our professional responsibilities and personal well-being. The future of work-life equilibrium holds the key to a more fulfilling and sustainable way of living, both during and beyond the pandemic.

The COVID-19 crisis has forced us to reevaluate our priorities and rethink the traditional norms of work. Many individuals have found themselves working remotely, blurring the lines between their professional and personal lives. While this shift initially presented its challenges, it has also opened up new opportunities for creating a more harmonious work-life balance.

One of the key aspects of the future of work-life equilibrium is the recognition that productivity does not solely depend on the number of hours spent at work. Instead, it emphasizes the importance of setting clear boundaries, managing time effectively, and focusing on meaningful outcomes. This shift towards a results-oriented approach allows individuals to be productive while also taking care of their personal needs and well-being.

Moreover, the future of work-life equilibrium involves embracing flexibility and autonomy in our work arrangements. The pandemic has proven that many roles can be successfully performed remotely, offering individuals the freedom to choose where and when they work. This newfound flexibility enables people to better integrate their professional and personal lives, leading to increased satisfaction and overall well-being.

However, achieving work-life equilibrium requires a collective effort from both employers and employees. Organizations must prioritize employee well-being and implement policies that promote a healthy work-life balance. This may include offering flexible work hours, encouraging regular breaks, and providing resources for mental health support. By creating a supportive work environment, employers can foster a culture that values work-life equilibrium and empowers their employees to thrive.

For individuals, the future of work-life equilibrium calls for a proactive approach to self-care and personal development. It involves setting boundaries, practicing self-discipline, and nurturing healthy habits. This may include establishing a dedicated workspace, scheduling regular breaks, and engaging in activities that promote physical and mental well-being. By prioritizing self-care, individuals can better manage the demands of their work and personal life, ultimately leading to greater satisfaction and happiness.

In conclusion, the future of work-life equilibrium holds immense potential for creating a more fulfilling and sustainable way of living. By embracing flexibility, setting boundaries, and prioritizing well-being, individuals and organizations can navigate the challenges of the pandemic while also building a foundation for a future where work and life are in balance. It is up to each and every one of us to take charge of our own work-life equilibrium and create a brighter future for ourselves and those around us.

Long-term strategies for maintaining equilibrium post-pandemic

The COVID-19 pandemic has upended our lives in countless ways, creating a new normal that has forced us to adapt and find ways to maintain equilibrium amidst the chaos. As we navigate the challenges of being productive during a pandemic, it becomes crucial to develop long-term strategies to ensure that we can continue to thrive even after the crisis subsides.

One of the most effective long-term strategies for maintaining equilibrium post-pandemic is to prioritize self-care. Taking care of ourselves physically, mentally, and emotionally is essential for overall well-being and productivity. This can include establishing a regular exercise routine, practicing mindfulness and meditation, engaging in hobbies or activities that bring joy, and seeking support from loved ones or professionals when needed. By investing in our own well-being, we can build resilience and better cope with future challenges.

Another key strategy is to embrace flexibility and adaptability. The pandemic has taught us the importance of being able to pivot and adjust our plans when circumstances change. By cultivating a mindset of adaptability, we can better navigate uncertainties and setbacks that may arise post-pandemic. This can involve being open to new opportunities, developing new skills, and seeking out diverse perspectives to broaden our horizons.

Building a strong support network is also crucial for maintaining equilibrium in the long run. Surrounding ourselves with individuals who uplift and inspire us can provide a sense of community and help us stay motivated. Whether it's colleagues, friends, or mentors, having a support system that understands our unique challenges and goals is invaluable. Additionally, seeking out professional networks and communities that align with our interests can offer opportunities for growth and collaboration.

Lastly, it is essential to establish healthy boundaries and prioritize work-life integration. The pandemic has blurred the lines between work and personal life, making it challenging to disconnect and recharge. Setting clear boundaries around work hours, creating designated spaces for work and relaxation, and scheduling regular breaks are all vital for maintaining a sense of equilibrium. By consciously integrating work and personal life in a balanced way, we can avoid burnout and ensure long-term well-being.

In conclusion, as we strive to be productive during the pandemic, it is crucial to develop long-term strategies for maintaining equilibrium post-pandemic. Prioritizing self-care, embracing flexibility, building a support network, and establishing healthy boundaries are all vital components of achieving work-life equilibrium for everyone. By implementing these strategies, we can not only navigate the challenges of the pandemic but also thrive in the post-pandemic world.

Recognizing the evolving needs of a diverse workforce

In the wake of the global pandemic, society as a whole has been forced to adapt to a new way of living and working. The impact of these changes has been particularly significant for individuals in the workforce, who have had to navigate the challenges of remote work, increased stress levels, and the blurring of boundaries between work and personal life. As we strive to achieve work-life equilibrium for everyone, it is crucial to recognize the evolving needs of a diverse workforce.

One of the key aspects of recognizing these evolving needs is understanding that every individual's experience during the pandemic has been unique. People come from different backgrounds, have varying responsibilities, and face distinct challenges. For some, the transition to remote work has been seamless, allowing for increased productivity and flexibility. However, for others, it has been a source of added stress and isolation.

To address these diverse needs, organizations must adopt a more inclusive approach to work. This involves acknowledging the different circumstances that employees may be facing and providing appropriate support and resources. For example, companies can offer flexible work schedules to accommodate individuals who are juggling caregiving responsibilities or dealing with health issues. Additionally, investing in mental health initiatives and promoting work-life balance can go a long way in supporting the well-being of all employees.

Furthermore, recognizing the evolving needs of a diverse workforce also means embracing diversity and inclusion in the workplace. This includes creating an environment where individuals of all backgrounds feel valued, respected, and included. By fostering a culture of inclusivity, organizations can tap into the unique perspectives and talents that a diverse workforce brings, ultimately driving innovation and success.

In order to be productive during the pandemic, it is essential to acknowledge and address the evolving needs of a diverse workforce. By doing so, organizations can create an environment that supports the well-being of all employees and ensures that everyone has an equal opportunity to thrive. As we continue to navigate the challenges of the pandemic, let us strive for work-life equilibrium that is inclusive and beneficial for everyone.

Advocating for a sustainable work-life equilibrium for everyone

Subchapter: Advocating for a Sustainable Work-Life Equilibrium for Everyone

Introduction:
In the midst of the ongoing pandemic, the concept of work-life balance has become increasingly challenging to achieve. Many individuals find themselves struggling to maintain productivity while juggling personal responsibilities, remote work, and the constant fear and uncertainty brought on by the pandemic. This subchapter aims to address the importance of advocating for a sustainable work-life equilibrium for everyone, offering practical strategies to enhance productivity during these challenging times.

1. Acknowledging the Importance of Work-Life Equilibrium:
Work-life equilibrium refers to the delicate balance between professional commitments and personal well-being. It is crucial to recognize the significance of this equilibrium, as it directly impacts our mental health, overall happiness, and productivity levels. The pandemic has further emphasized the need for individuals to find harmony in their lives and prioritize their well-being.

2. Understanding the Challenges of Being Productive During a Pandemic:
The pandemic has introduced a myriad of challenges that can hinder productivity. Factors such as increased anxiety, blurred boundaries between work and personal life, limited social interactions, and lack of motivation can significantly impact our ability to stay focused and

efficient. Identifying these challenges is the first step towards finding effective solutions.

3. Strategies for Achieving Sustainable Work-Life Equilibrium:
a. Establishing Boundaries: Set clear boundaries between work and personal life by defining specific working hours, creating a designated workspace, and communicating these boundaries with colleagues and family members.
b. Prioritizing Self-Care: Engage in activities that promote well-being, such as regular exercise, meditation, and maintaining a healthy lifestyle. Taking care of yourself is essential for sustained productivity.
c. Time Management Techniques: Utilize effective time management techniques such as the Pomodoro Technique, time blocking, and creating to-do lists to enhance productivity and maintain focus.
d. Effective Communication: Maintain open and transparent communication with colleagues and supervisors. Discuss workload, deadlines, and any challenges you may be facing to ensure a healthy work environment.
e. Embracing Flexibility: Embrace the flexibility that remote work offers. Schedule breaks and allow yourself time to recharge. Flexibility allows for a healthier work-life equilibrium.

Conclusion:
Advocating for a sustainable work-life equilibrium during the pandemic is crucial for maintaining productivity and overall well-being. By acknowledging the challenges and implementing practical strategies, individuals can navigate the uncertainties of the current situation while finding balance and contentment in their lives. Remember, achieving work-life equilibrium is not a luxury but a

necessity for everyone, and by prioritizing it, we can create a future where productivity and personal well-being coexist harmoniously.

Conclusion: Achieving Work-Life Equilibrium: A Journey of Balance and Growth

In the midst of the global pandemic, our lives have been upended in ways we never could have anticipated. The lines between work and personal life have blurred, leaving many of us feeling overwhelmed and struggling to find a sense of balance. However, it is possible to achieve work-life equilibrium even in these challenging times. It is a journey that requires conscious effort, self-reflection, and a commitment to growth.

Throughout this book, we have explored the concept of work-life equilibrium and its importance in maintaining our well-being and productivity during the pandemic. We have discussed practical strategies to help us navigate the new normal and make the most of our time and energy. Now, as we conclude this journey, let us reflect on the key principles that can guide us towards achieving work-life equilibrium:

1. Prioritize self-care: Taking care of ourselves is not a luxury; it is a necessity. When we prioritize self-care, we are better equipped to handle the challenges that come our way. Make time for activities that rejuvenate you, such as exercise, meditation, or spending quality time with loved ones.

2. Set boundaries: Establish clear boundaries between work and personal life. Define specific work hours and create a designated workspace. Communicate these boundaries to your colleagues and loved ones, ensuring that everyone understands and respects them.

3. Manage time effectively: Time is a finite resource, and it is crucial to use it wisely. Prioritize tasks, eliminate distractions, and practice time-blocking to ensure you allocate time for both work and personal activities. Remember to schedule breaks to recharge and avoid burnout.

4. Foster open communication: Communication is key, especially during times of uncertainty. Maintain open lines of communication with your colleagues, managers, and loved ones. Express your needs and concerns, and be receptive to feedback. Effective communication helps build understanding and support in all areas of life.

5. Embrace flexibility: Flexibility is the cornerstone of work-life equilibrium. Embrace the idea that work can be done from different locations and at different times. Advocate for flexible work arrangements that suit your needs and enable a harmonious integration of work and personal life.

Remember, achieving work-life equilibrium is not a destination but an ongoing journey. It requires constant self-reflection, adaptation, and growth. As we navigate the challenges of the pandemic, let us approach this journey with patience, resilience, and a commitment to our well-being. By prioritizing ourselves, setting boundaries, managing time effectively, fostering open communication, and embracing flexibility, we can find balance and unlock our full potential.

The pandemic may have presented us with a paradox, but it has also given us an opportunity for personal and professional growth. Let us seize this opportunity and strive for work-life equilibrium, not just during these challenging times, but for the rest of our lives. Together, we can create a future where everyone can thrive, both personally and professionally, no matter the circumstances.

In this book, "The Pandemic Paradox: Achieving Work-Life Equilibrium for Everyone," we have explored the challenges and opportunities that the pandemic has brought upon us. We have delved into the importance of finding a balance between work and personal life, especially in the midst of these uncertain times. Now, as we conclude this journey, let us reflect on the valuable lessons we have learned and the steps we can take to achieve work-life equilibrium.

The pandemic presented us with a unique opportunity to reevaluate our priorities and redefine what it means to be productive. We discovered that productivity is not solely measured by the number of tasks accomplished, but also by the quality of our work and the well-being of our mind and body. As we navigated the uncharted waters of remote work and social distancing, we learned to adapt and find new ways to stay connected, both professionally and personally.

One of the key takeaways from this book is the importance of setting boundaries. We must establish clear boundaries between work and personal life to prevent burnout and maintain a healthy work-life balance. By creating designated workspaces and defining working hours, we can maintain a sense of structure and separate our professional and personal responsibilities.

Another vital aspect of achieving work-life equilibrium is self-care. Taking care of ourselves physically, mentally, and emotionally is crucial, especially during challenging times. We explored various self-care practices such as exercise, meditation, and maintaining healthy relationships. These practices not only enhance our overall well-being but also contribute to our productivity and ability to cope with stress.

Furthermore, we discovered the significance of effective time management. By prioritizing tasks, setting realistic goals, and embracing flexibility, we can optimize our productivity and reduce the feeling of overwhelm. We also explored the benefits of incorporating breaks and downtime into our schedules, allowing us to recharge and return to work with renewed focus and creativity.

As we conclude this book, we want to emphasize that achieving work-life equilibrium is not a one-time accomplishment, but rather an ongoing journey of growth and adaptation. It requires continuous self-reflection, adjustment, and a commitment to our well-being. By implementing the strategies and insights shared in this book, we can create a harmonious synergy between our work and personal lives, leading to a more fulfilling and balanced existence.

Remember, you have the power to shape your own work-life equilibrium. Embrace the lessons learned, prioritize your well-being, and embark on this journey of balance and growth. Together, we can navigate the challenges of the pandemic and emerge stronger, more resilient, and fulfilled individuals.

This book is dedicated to everyone seeking to find harmony amidst the chaos, and we hope that the insights shared within these pages will empower you to achieve work-life equilibrium and lead a fulfilling life during and beyond the pandemic.

www.ingramcontent.com/pod-product-compliance
Lightning Source LLC
LaVergne TN
LVHW051956060526
838201LV00059B/3674